Autism Friendly Training: First Responders

DR. LINDA BARBOA
JAN LUCK

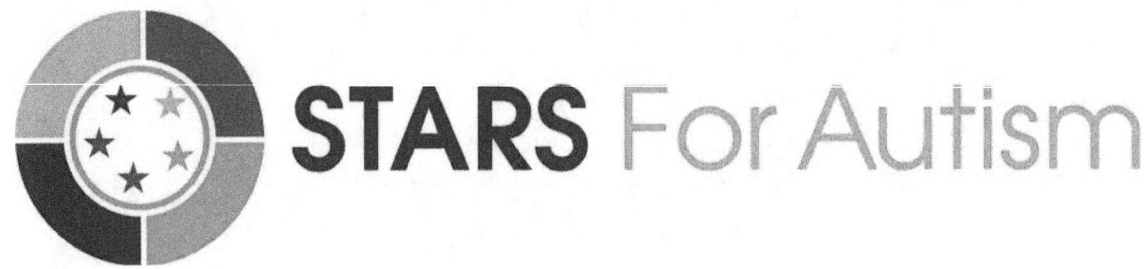

SUPPORT
TRAINING
AWARENESS
RESPECT
SERVICE

Copyright © 2016 Dr. Linda Barboa

All rights reserved.

No part of this publication may be reproduced, stored in a retrieval system or transmitted in any way, by any means, electronic, mechanical, photocopy, or otherwise without the prior permission of the author, except as provided by USA copyright law.

The information in this book is meant to supplement, not replace, proper first responder training. The authors and the presenters are not medical physicians, and do not represent themselves as such. The information presented is solely designed to present possible complications in a medical situation which may be complicated by autism.

ISBN-10: 1539547981

ISBN-13: 978-1539547983

Autism friendly……

means being aware of social engagement

and environmental factors

affecting people on the autism spectrum

with modifications to communication methods

and physical space

to better suit individual's unique and special needs.[i]

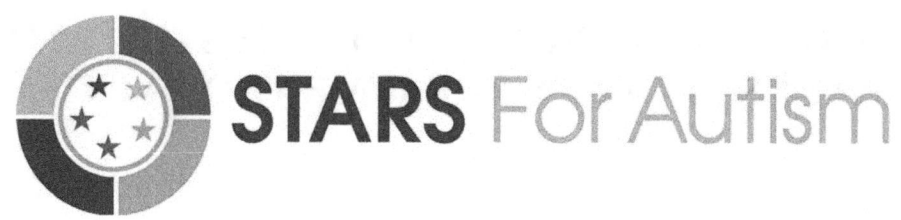

WHY DO FIRST RESPONDERS NEED TO KNOW ABOUT AUTISM?

The Center for Disease Control and Prevention (CDC) currently estimates that 1 in 68 children has autism, with the rate being 1 in every 42 boys. The identified rate is five times higher in boys than girls. It is one of the fastest growing developmental disabilities in the United States. Autism affects people of all races, nationalities and social classes. Autism is estimated to currently occur in 3.5 million Americans, so it is likely that you will have association with people on the spectrum. With the current statistics, it is safe to say that there are people living with autism in virtually every city in America. It has been stated that people with autism are more likely than their typical peers to require the services of a first responder at some point in their lives. If you have a career as a first responder we can assume that you will find yourself treating an individual on the spectrum at some point. The more that you understand about this complex disorder and prepare yourself for the eventuality, the more successful your encounters will be.

WHAT IS AUTISM?

Autism is a complex disorder. As we go through our everyday lives, our brains continually collect information about the world around us through our senses (including vision, hearing, smell, touch and taste). In autism, the senses may be over or under processing the incoming stimuli. People with autism are not able to make sense of the incoming sensory information. The issues may vary throughout a person's lifetime, or even day to day. Autism affects the ability to communicate, any or all of the senses, social abilities, and behavior.

WHAT IS THE ROLE OF THE 911 SYSTEM IN THE EMERGENCY TREATMENT OF AUTISM?

In many places around the country, the 911 system is the front line in meeting the needs at an emergency. Dispatchers are highly trained to record important data and to dispense that data to those responding. A person dialing 911 from locations where that service is available will be connected to emergency management. Some 911 service areas use a voluntary special needs registry to identify homes of persons with a variety of special needs, including autism. In those areas, if a call comes in to the 911 dispatcher, the information is automatically relayed about the special needs if the patron has signed up in advance. This allows the responders to know in advance what barriers they may face. Caregivers of individuals with autism may have installed extra locks or bars on doors if elopement is an issue. The first responder may be coming into a situation where a child may bolt, or where there could be communication difficulties. The responder may be alerted if the resident is prone to bolting, or does not respond to verbal directives. If the patient or another person in the home has autism, the first responder will have a more successful entry if he is able to get that information in advance. The responders might decide to avoid use of their emergency sirens and lights which could cause escalation of an incident if a person with autism is involved. A quieter, less visual approach could avoid added troubles.

WHAT ARE THE MAIN CHALLENGES ASSOCIATED WITH AUTISM?

The core features of autism include:
- Communication struggles
- Sensory issues
- Difficulty in social interactions
- Unusual behaviors

HOW ARE COMMUNICATION SKILLS AFFECTED?

Communication is our most basic connection to others in our world. When the ability to communicate effectively is missing, it interferes with a full and happy life. Although some people with autism may have advanced language skills, others may be severely language delayed. It is important that first responders remember that just because a person is non-verbal does not mean that they cannot understand what you are saying. It is common for individuals with autism to have receptive (understanding) skills far above their ability to express themselves. Communication skills may be affected in many ways including:

- May have lack of a social "filter"- they say what they think although the comment may be inappropriate or hurtful.
- May be delayed in language development.
- May remain basically nonverbal.
- May repeat words, phrases or entire paragraphs that they have heard before.
- May speak in a flat tone of voice.
- May have difficulty constructing sentences.
- May use some basic sign language or an electronic communication device.

COMMUNICATION TIPS FOR FIRST RESPONDERS

Sensory processing is often delayed in people on the autism spectrum. This includes neurologically processing what is being heard. When you speak to him, it may take him more time than expected to process and understand what you are saying. Give him time to think about what you are saying and time to provide a response. If you keep asking questions or giving directions in rapid succession, he will just get more and more confused. Be patient. Other tips that will assist your communication are:

- Say what you mean. Avoid idioms and figures of speech.
- Do not tease or joke - this person will take what you say literally.
- If the person seems to not understand what you are saying, change your wording. Don't simply repeat the exact same words, and don't speak louder. People with autism very often have a variety of communication issues that make it difficult not only to speak, but to understand what you are telling them.
- Keep directions simple. Giving directions with many steps may be confusing.
- The person may not understand facial expressions or body language, including pointing.
- The person must be given very direct instructions. He often will not understand an indirect instruction. For example, do not say, "I need to look in your mouth now." Rather, say, "Open your mouth." Rather than saying, "I can't wrap this bandage on your leg while you are kicking," Say, "Hold your leg still."
- Explain the use of your flashlight, tongue depressor, and other medical tools, perhaps letting them touch the tool before you use it with the patient. The person may think the flashlight is fire rather than merely a small light, and may have a

violent reaction to the sight of it.
- Give instructions as a directive rather than as a question. Rather than saying, "Can you open your mouth for me?" say, "Open your mouth." They may not recognize the question as a directive, but may merely think you are asking them a question.
- If there is a behavioral issue involved, communication is your first strategy to de-escalate the situation.
- Communicating with the caregiver will give you vital information about the person's abilities and how their reactions may be different from a typical person's behaviors.

WHAT DO FIRST RESPONDERS NEED TO UNDERSTAND ABOUT FAMILIES?

- Families are often stressed with the challenges of autism in the home and school.
- Estimates show that the cost to raise a child with autism range from $1.4 million to $2.5 million with medical costs, special schooling, and therapies being costly.
- Children with autism often have other medical complications adding to the stress.
- Families of children with autism are often sleep deprived, as the children often suffer from sleep disorders.
- The stress of autism often takes a toll on the family as a whole.
- Taking an individual with autism out into the community can be difficult and stressful for the family. People sometimes stare, fail to understand behaviors that occur, or make hurtful comments to the family.
- The time and resources that a family directs toward the child with autism may take away from a typical childhood for the siblings.

HOW SHOULD A PROVIDER COMMUNICATE WITH THE CAREGIVER OF A CHILD WITH AUTISM?

- Do not give unsolicited advice about discipline, diets, treatments or "cures."
- Do not comment on the child looking "normal." Do comment about the child's appearance as you would with any other child, such as, "Your hair looks pretty today" or, "I like that blue shirt."
- Do not ask if the child is a genius, a savant or has special skills. Do comment as you would with any other child, such as, "Are you a Cardinals fan?"

- Do not ask what caused the autism.
- Do not say you know exactly what the parent is going through.
- Do not say, "God never gives us more than we can handle" or "You must be such a special person."
- LISTEN to what the caregiver tells you about the patient with autism. The family is the 24/7 team and knows the person better than anyone else does. They can tell you what calms him, what agitates him, and how to handle him.

WHAT DO THE SENSES HAVE TO DO WITH AUTISM?

Distorted sensory perception is a major part of autism. The way a person with autism perceives the world around him is different from the way that others get information from the environment. One or more of these senses may be affected:

- Vision - Confused sensory processing of visual stimuli may result in the person either being too sensitive to light and other visual stimuli, or not sensitive enough. Eye contact may be disturbing to the person. Do not demand that he look you in the eye. He may be confused or upset by rapid movements in his line of vision, or random movements. Professionals attempting to treat a person with autism may find it helpful to approach gently, and explain what movements you are making.

- Hearing - Confused sensory processing can result in the person being either too sensitive to the sounds in the environment or not sensitive enough. Professionals may find it helpful to move to a quiet area to reduce the person's agitation. If you are treating a person who seems to not be responding to your voice, do not increase to a shouting level. Continue to use a calm voice, possibly using different words. When a person does not respond to commands, do not assume that he cannot hear.

- Taste - Confused sensory processing may distort his perception of things he tastes. Items may seem tasteless or far too intense. Distorted sense of taste sometimes results in the person ingesting a harmful substance, such as poisonous mixtures.

- Smell - Confused sensory processing of things he smells may result in those odors being far too intense or simply lacking. He may be repulsed by the smell of items that we normally do not notice, or he may be drawn to noxious odors.

- Feeling & Touch - Confused sensory processing can result in not feeling things enough or feeling them too strongly. This may apply to a touch, clothing, or things as light as air. The feel of a band aid or bandage may be upsetting to him, as he might feel it far more intensely than a typical person would. Often a light touch is more disturbing to him than a firm touch. His reaction to warm or cool rooms may be exaggerated. He may want to strip his clothing off if he feels extremely warm. Items such as gauze or bandages may elicit a strong reaction if it is averse to him. It is highly important for first responders to understand that a person with autism may not react to pain in the way that others do. He may scream in pain at a touch that others would barely even notice. On the other hand, he may not even seem to feel a quite severe wound. Not reacting to a severe injury, combined with not being able to communicate his needs complicates the treatment. They may even laugh, hum, sing, or remove clothing as a response to pain.

Along with the five senses discussed above, which are the five senses commonly learned about in school, there are three additional senses that may be affected in people with autism.

- Vestibular (the sense of knowing where his body is in relation to the Earth). Poor vestibular processing results in poor balance and coordination. People with autism may have a severe reaction of claustrophobia if they are put into a small space, or if there are a lot of people crowding around.

- Proprioception (the sensory system that informs the person about the position of his body in relation to the space around him). Poor proprioceptive processing results in clumsiness, and lack of coordination. Be aware that this person may regularly have bruises due to bumping into objects and falling. The large number of bruises must be differentiated from abuse by a caregiver.

- Interoception (the sense of what is happening in one's own body). Throughout each person's body are many receptors. The body sends information to the brain to allow us to make sense of these messages, such as hunger, the need to go to the bathroom, itch, pain, body temperature, nausea, and other bodily signals. Interoception also allows us to feel our emotions. People with autism do not receive these signals in the typical way and may have confusions about the signals their body sends the brain. They may laugh inappropriately, or show sleep or eating disturbances.

One or more of the senses may be affected. This can vary from day to day- or even minute to minute. Many of the behaviors you notice may be the person's efforts to *avoid* a certain sensation or to *seek* more sensory input from the world around him.

HOW ARE SOCIAL SKILLS AFFECTED?

Appropriate social interactions are important for a happy and productive life. Forging friendships and having good relationships with others is dependent on successful social interactions. People on the autism spectrum may exhibit some or all of these social difficulties:

- Difficulty with eye contact
- Inability to interpret facial expression or other gestures
- Poor social or emotional connections
- Little or no interest in others
- Lack the ability to see things from another's point of view
- Lack of understanding humor
- Very literal thinking
- Extreme attachments to a toy or another object
- May play with toys in unusual or unexpected ways
- May be afraid of things they need not fear and not fear things that most people fear
- May shun or crave physical contact with others
- Needs predictability and routine - change is difficult
- May do unusual actions repeatedly
- May seem to want to be alone - withdrawn
- May have a hard time interacting with others
- May have outbursts due to sensory or communicative struggles

WHAT BEHAVIORS MAY BE ASSOCIATED WITH AUTISM?

Although the characteristics vary widely from person to person there is a set of characteristics that are common in this group of people. Behavior is an attempt to communicate. A person's behaviors are his way of communicating his needs, his sensory overloads and his frustrations. Behaviors you may observe in people with autism include:

- Withdrawal
- Aggression due to problems in communication and frustrations about the sensory input he receives from the environment
- Self-stimulation such as rocking, jumping, flapping the hands, humming or chanting

- Meltdowns
- Unusual pattern of interests, such as high interest in one topic, like dinosaurs, vacuums, or the solar system
- May need order, "sameness," and extreme organization
- May have preoccupation with certain behaviors, have odd routines or rituals
- May have unusual mannerisms
- May lack appropriate response to pain
- May laugh inappropriately
- May lack fear of danger and may be afraid of things not typically feared
- May have odd or repetitive play
- May not like touch or may seem not to feel it
- May have difficulty in regulating emotions
- May be drawn to water when wandering or running

WHAT MODIFICATIONS MIGHT I MAKE IN MY EXAM OF THIS PATIENT?

Using the information given to you by the 911 dispatcher or the caregiver, modify your approach as needed. Be prepared for unexpected reactions to any sensory stimuli. It may be comforting to an agitated patient to wrap him in a blanket. He may resist any type of rescue activity. It may be helpful to demonstrate each action on another person so that the individual understands what you will do to him. It is sometimes helpful to perform the exam in a distal to proximal manner. During the exam be very aware of the possibility of positional asphyxia as many people on the autism spectrum have poor core body strength.

WHY IS AUTISM CALLED A SPECTRUM DISORDER?

You will hear autism referred to as a "spectrum disorder." This means that each person's abilities and behaviors might fall along a very wide range from high functioning to low functioning. The outward signs vary greatly from person to person. Autism spectrum disorder is often abbreviated ASD.

HOW IS AUTISM DIAGNOSED?

There is no medical test for autism. Specially trained physicians, neurologists, and psychologists diagnose autism through behavioral observations and analysis. Some of the behaviors that are associated with autism may be the result of another illness or cultural problem. These behaviors do not always indicate autism. The diagnostic process is complicated and extensive. Please do not "second guess" the medical professionals who have given the diagnosis.

DOES AUTISM RUN IN FAMILIES?

There does seem to be an indication that it is more prevalent in some families. Even though autism runs in some families, we can't say it is "inherited."

WHAT CAUSES AUTISM?

There are many theories as to the cause of autism and why it is increasing at such a fast rate. It is suspected that there may be a genetic factor and an environmental factor, although no cause has been proven. The important thing to know is that it is not caused by the parents' behavior. Theories about autism being caused by emotionally cold parents have been long disproven. You may see claims made on almost a daily basis of various causes and links to autism, but at this point there is not a known cause- just many theories.

HOW IS PHYSICAL CONTACT AFFECTED?

Many people with autism avoid physical contact with others. The touch from another person may actually be painful if their sense of touch is overly developed. There are others who are perfectly fine with having someone touch them, especially if they are the one to initiate the physical contact. Often a stronger, firm touch is more accepted by him than a light, feathery touch, which may feel painful. You may encounter other people with autism who crave physical contact and may rush to hug you very strongly.

IS A MELTDOWN JUST A TEMPER TANTRUM?

A meltdown is different from a tantrum. Temper tantrums are thrown by a child who wants something such as a toy, or wants to avoid something, such as chores. When he gets what he wants, the tantrum ends. He relies on having an audience, and normally will not continue the tantrum otherwise. A meltdown, on the other hand, is a very intense reaction to being overwhelmed or overstressed. This does not end by reaching a goal, but more likely ends by fatigue setting in. A meltdown is not dependent on having an audience. The person may truly need help to regain control. While a temper tantrum normally lasts a few minutes, a meltdown can continue for several hours.

Remember that the parent has been through this before and knows the child best. While it is acceptable to calmly ask the parent if there is anything you can do to help, please respect the parent's decision. If she tells you that she has the situation under control, allow the parent to work through the meltdown. Do not make judgmental comments or give disapproving looks. If there is a quiet area that the parent may take the child to while they work through the sensory overload, offer that to the parent.

ARE ALL PEOPLE WITH AUTISM GENIUSES?

Just as people who do not have autism exhibit skills all along the range of intellectual abilities, the same applies to those with autism. Intellectual skills may range from intellectually challenged to gifted.

WHAT IS ASPERGER'S SYNDROME?

Asperger's Syndrome is technically one form of autism, on the higher functioning end of the autism spectrum. People with Asperger's usually have difficulties with social situations but not with language development. They are often very literal thinkers and struggle to understand humor, figures of speech, sarcasm and words with multiple meanings. They may be rigid in their schedules, and often have sensory issues. People with Asperger's usually function well in daily life and in society even though they struggle with social expectations and understandings.

WHAT SHOULD I TELL PEOPLE IF THEY ASK MY OPINION AS TO WHETHER THEIR CHILD HAS AUTISM?

Tell them a good place to start is by talking to their pediatrician. They should make this contact as soon as possible. Their doctor can give them the information needed to contact services for diagnosis and treatment. A helpful book to read at that point is *Stars in Her Eyes; Navigating the Maze of Childhood Autism* by Barboa and Obrey (2014). This book will lead them by the hand through the diagnosis process and into intervention decisions. Urge them to not fear the diagnosis, as that can be the key to unlock many doors, such as educational services and financial assistance. It is also helpful for them talk to others who have children on the spectrum, as those people can lead them to resources and services in your area.

CAN PEOPLE WITH AUTISM BECOME PRODUCTIVE MEMBERS OF SOCIETY?

High-functioning people on the spectrum are likely to be very successful in college and excel in the fields of science and medicine. Traits commonly noted in people with autism, such as a strong need for structure and intense focus on interests, can be an assets in the work force in many different fields. Adaptations and modifications are often needed, along with special training for both the individual and the employer. Although they may need extensive assistance, most people on the autism spectrum can become contributing members of society.

Adults with autism often have some special needs. Each person's needs will differ, but this is a list of needs that many have in common:

- Vocational training based on the person's strengths and interests
- Job opportunities where the employer and co-workers have been trained to understand the challenges of autism
- Group homes, supervised apartments, or other alternate living arrangements
- Recreational and social opportunities where they can feel accepted and not judged

Autism involves continuous, lifelong progress in all areas, including social awareness, learning new skills and finding new enjoyable experiences. What do adults with autism need to be successful as adults? They need compassionate, continuous support in areas that others take for granted. They need understanding from the community as they try hard to lead fulfilling lives.

WHAT DOES IT MEAN TO BE "AUTISM FRIENDLY?"

Autism friendly means that you are aware of social engagement and of the possible environmental factors which might affect people on the **autism spectrum**. You are aware of possible ways to modify your communication methods and the physical environment to better suit each individual's special needs.

WHAT DO THESE TERMS AND ACRONYMS MEAN?

As you navigate the maze of autism you will find yourself dealing with some terms and acronyms which may be unfamiliar to you. This guide will give you a brief explanation of those which are among the most commonly used.

AACs: Augmentative and alternative communication devices. Electronic devices used to speak for the mostly non-verbal person.

ABA: Applied Behavior Analysis. A structured program that many parents feel is highly successful. Used by trained professionals.

ADD: Attention Deficit Disorder.

ADHD: Hyperactivity added to ADD.

Alerting stimulants: Things in the environment which make the child more alert or more awake.

Aromatherapy: Some smells may be invigorating while others may be soothing to the child.

Articulation: The way we pronounce our words.

ASD: Autism Spectrum Disorder.

Asperger's Syndrome: A form of autism which is characterized by social awkwardness.

Aspie: An affectionate term for a person with Asperger's.

Attachment: A person with autism may become highly attached to a random object or toy.

Auditory: The sense of hearing.

Auditory processing: The system by which the brain makes sense of the sounds we hear.

Auditory sensitivities: Child may be overly or under sensitive to sounds.

AutPlay ® Therapy: Developed by Dr. Robert Grant, this method combines behavioral and developmental techniques.

Avoidance behavior: A learned coping mechanism in which the person with autism withdraws from a situation to escape some stimuli that is aversive to him.

Babbling: Early speech sounds such as, "mama" or "dada" which are normal speech productions for a baby.

Behavioral: Any action that is not purely reflexive.

Biomedical: Treatments that address physical symptoms.

BIP: Behavior Intervention Plan implemented by a school.

Brushing: A therapy technique used to produce a calming, sensory organizing effect.

Calming skills: Persons with autism may need to be taught techniques to calm themselves.

Casein: A protein in dairy that may have an adverse effect on some people.

ChoicesChat© short simple chats you have with a child about choices he has made, and what may be a better choice the next time.[ii]   First identified by Barboa and Obrey in 2015.

Co-morbidities: Other diagnoses that occur along with the primary issue.

Coping skills: People learn to cope with unpleasant situations in a variety of ways. Some coping skills are negative and others are positive.

Cycling: Some children will learn a skill, lose the skill, and need to re-learn it, in a cyclical fashion.

Deep pressure: A therapy technique for calming and making sense of incoming sensations.

Discrete Trial Training: A highly structured method of teaching used by highly trained professionals.

DSM: Diagnostic and Statistical Manual of Mental Disorders, used as criteria for diagnosing disorders.

Early Intervention: Identification and treatment that begins in early childhood.

Echolalia: Repetition of a sound, word or phrase that the child has heard another person say.

Expressive Language: The language that the person can actually produce.

Flapping: A sensory stimulating activity in which a child flaps his hands or arms.

Gluten: A protein in some grains which has an adverse effect on some people.

Gustatory: The sense of taste.

Hyperacusis: An abnormal reaction to sound.

Hyperlexia: A splinter skill of being able to decode reading words at a higher level than he can comprehend.

Hypersensitive: Overly sensitive.

Hyposensitive: Too low sensitivity.

IDEA: Individuals with Disabilities Education Act. Federal law guarantees a free and appropriate education for all children.

IEP: Individual Education Plan (or Program). Plan developed by the parent and the school to provide for the child's educational needs.

Incidental learning: Learning that happens informally.

Inclusion: When special education services are brought into the regular classroom to individualize instruction.

Joint attention: Communication between two people.

Learned helplessness: When we provide too much help for a child rather than expecting him to do things for himself, he will take longer to learn that skill.

Mainstreaming: The process of integrating your child into a typical classroom.

Melatonin: A plant product sold as a supplement.

Meltdowns: Overstimulation which results in the child being overwhelmed and losing control.

Occupational therapy: Can help balance out sensory perceptions.

Olfactory: Sense of smell.

Parental rights: In the educational system these are designated by law.

PECS®: Picture Exchange Communication System. Technique used by specially trained professions, using small pictures to communicate.

Perseveration: Repetition of a movement or sound.

PDD: Pervasive Developmental Disorder. May be used interchangeably with the word "autism" or may refer to a child who has some of the characteristics, but not all.

Pica: Desire to eat non-edible objects such as dirt.

Pragmatics: The social aspect of speech, such as greetings and conversational skills.

Predictability: People with autism usually have a deep need to know the schedule.

PrepChat©: Developed by Barboa and Obrey, this is a simplified chat that you have with the child to discuss and upcoming event and prepare him for what he will encounter.

Proprioception: The sensory system that informs your child of the position of his body in relation to the space around him.

QR codes©: Patches registered online which can be sewn into clothing to be scanned to reveal the child's important identifying information. Developed by "If I Need Help," a non-profit organization.

Quiet rooms: Rooms in a public place such as a theater or church where parents or teachers can calm children who are getting overwhelmed.

Receptive language: The vocabulary that a person can understand as opposed to what he produces.

Reinforcers: Rewards given for behaviors or tasks completed.

Respite: Help given by another to take care of the person who has special needs to give the parent or guardian a break.

Rett's Disorder: A genetic disorder which results in behaviors of autism.

Rituals: Routines or activities that the person seems compelled to perform, such as flicking the light on and off multiple times.

Scaffolding: Refers to the assistance given to a child in learning to complete a task. Like a painter standing on a scaffold to reach higher than he could otherwise, teaching techniques help the child achieve higher levels of learning.

Scripting: People repeating segments of conversations or television shows they have heard.

Self-injurious behaviors: Behaviors by a person to willfully inflict harm on himself.

Self-stimulation: When a person creates stimuli or sensory input for himself, such as rocking, flapping, or spinning.

Sensory input: The stimulation received through the environment.

Sensory integration: Processing information received from the body and the environment.

Social referencing: When a child looks to others for approval or acknowledgement.

Splinter skills: Talents that are far above the rest of the person's abilities.

Stimming/ self-stim: See "self-stimulation."

Stimuli/ stimulus: Anything that creates a reaction in the person.

Tactile: The sense of touch.

Tactile defensiveness: Not wanting to be touched.

Task analysis: Breaking down a job into its smaller steps.

Transitioning: Changing from one activity to the next. This is often a special challenge for children on the spectrum.

Vestibular activities: Jumping, rocking, balancing, swinging, etc.

Weighted vests: A calming strategy used under the direction of an occupational therapist.

WHAT MORE CAN I DO TO HELP?

Many communities across the country now have a special needs 911 registry. Families can fill out a simple form, and file it with the 911 managers, informing the first responders of the disability of a family member. When a responder is dispatched to the listed address, the dispatcher can give verbal information that will prepare the responder to the special circumstances in the home they are about to encounter. They can be informed that a non-verbal person with autism is in the home and may not respond to directions. They may be told that the child in the home is prone to bolting when the door is opened, and they can be prepared to be cautions. If your community has a special needs registry for the 911 system, encourage people to sign up with that service.

Be alert for either commercial or handwritten signs or stickers that parents may have used to notify first responders that a person with autism is in the car or in the home, and may have communication or behavior issues.

Seat belt notification cuffs are becoming more available. Watch for seat belt identifiers or various styles or colors with may be used to alert you of the special needs.

If you wish to support the work of an organization which is dedicated to improving education about autism, your efforts or your cash donations are highly appreciated. STARS for Autism is a nonprofit organization. Its mission is to network, collaborate, promote and support efforts, training, awareness, respect, and service for individuals and families with autism. Stars for Autism provides education and literature to teach people about autism. If you would like to support this effort, please visit our website for more information.

www.Stars4autism.org

and please enjoy our Facebook page "Stars for Autism"

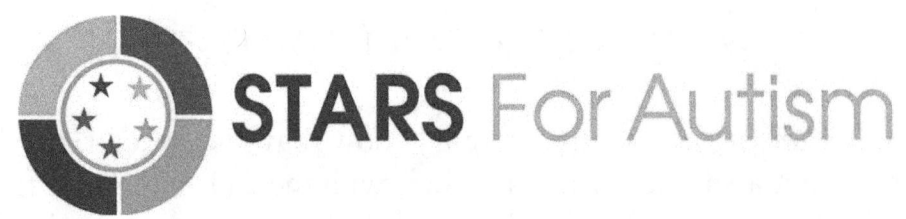

Helpful Books About Autism

Stars in Her Eyes; Navigating the Maze of Childhood Autism, by Dr. Linda Barboa and Elizabeth Obrey. Tate Publishing.

Tic Toc Autism Clock; A Guide to Your 24/7 Plan, by Elizabeth Obrey and Dr. Linda Barboa. Goldminds Publishing.

It's No Biggie; Autism in the Early Childhood Classroom, by Dr. Linda Barboa and Mary Lou Datema. Goldminds Publishing.

Steps: Forming a Disability Ministry, by Shelli Allen and Dr. Linda Barboa.

That Autism Mom's Guide to Homeschooling, by Shelli Allen.

Autplay® Therapy for Children and Adolescents on the Autism Spectrum: A Behavioral Play-Based Approach, by Dr. Robert Jason Grant.

Play-Based Interventions for Autism Spectrum Disorder and Other Developmental Disabilities, by Dr. Robert Jason Grant.

Autism Spectrum Disorder Workbook for Children, by Dr. Robert Jason Grant.

Positively Sensory, by Amy Stark Vaughn.

The Nuts and Bolts of Autism, by Dr. Linda Barboa and Jan Luck.

Children's Books

To help children understand autism, we recommend:

Albert is My Friend; Helping Children Understand Autism (also available in Spanish, German, and Dutch) by Jan Luck and Dr. Linda Barboa. Goldminds Publishing.

Albert Thinks About His Future by Jan Luck and Dr. Linda Barboa. Goldminds Publishing.

Albert Goes to School by Dr. Linda Barboa and Jan Luck.

Albert Goes to Church by Dr. Linda Barboa and Jan Luck.

Albert Goes to Camp by Dr. Linda Barboa and Jan Luck.

Albert Builds a Friend Ship by Jan Luck and Dr. Linda Barboa. Goldminds Publishing.

The Alien Logs of Super Jewels, by BK Bradshaw and Jaqi Bradshaw. Goldminds Publishing.

"AH-HA! Thoughts"

Use this page to jot down things you want to remember--

[i] https://en.wikipedia.org/wiki/Autism_spectrum_disorder
[ii] Barboa, L. and Obrey, E. *Tic Toc Autism Clock: A Guide to Your 24/7 Plan,* (USA: Goldminds Publishing, 2016).

www.ingramcontent.com/pod-product-compliance
Lightning Source LLC
Chambersburg PA
CBHW080646190526
45169CB00009B/3523